I0102160

Introduction to Yoga

- Weight Management Series

Volume 5

Excerpt from Adopting a healthy lifestyle (1-884711-34-0)

Introduction to Yoga
Weight Management Series

C.T. Pam

Copyright © 2013 by C. T. Pam

Published and printed in the United States by Innovative Publishers, Inc., Boston, Massachusetts.

Library of Congress Control Number: 2012955109

1-884711-52-9   978-1-884711-52-7 Paperback
Also available in the following formats
1-884711-53-7   978-1-884711-53-4 Kindle
1-884711-54-5   978-1-884711-54-1 Hardback
1-884711-55-3   978-1-884711-55-8 AudioBook
1-884711-56-1   978-1-884711-56-5 iBook
1-884711-57-X   978-1-884711-57-2 Nook

Designations used by companies to distinguish their products are often claimed as trademarks. In all instances where Innovative Publishers Inc. is aware of the claim, the product name appears in initial capital or all capital letters. Readers, however, should contact the appropriate companies for more complete information regarding trademarks and registration.

No part of this publication may be reproduced, stored in a retrieval system, or transmitted in any form or by any means, electronic, mechanical, photocopying, recording, scanning, or otherwise except as permitted under Section 107 or 108 of the 1976 United States Copyright Act, without either the prior written permission of the publisher, or authorization through payment of the appropriate per copy fee to the Copyright Clearance Center, 222 Rosewood Dr., Danvers, MA 01923, 978 – 750 – 8400, fax 978 – 646 – 8600, or on the web at www.copyright.com. Requests to the publisher for permission should be addressed to the Permissions Department, Innovative Publishers Inc., PO Box 300446, Boston, MA 02130, or online at http://innovative-publishers.com.

The information contained in this book is not intended to serve as a replacement for professional medical advice. Any use of the information in this book is that the reader's discretion. The author and the publisher specifically disclaim any and all liability arising directly or indirectly from the use or application of any information contained in this book. A healthcare professional should be consulted regarding your specific situation. For general information about our other products and services, please contact our customer care department within the United States. Specific contact information can be found online at http://innovative-publishers.com.

Printed in the United States of America

10 9 8 7 6 5 4 3 2 1   13 14 15 16

First edition, February 2013

All rights reserved under International and Pan-American
Copyright Conventions.

Limit of Liability/Disclaimer of Warranty: While the publisher and author have
used their best efforts in preparing this book, they make no representations or
warranties with respect to the accuracy or completeness of the contents of this
book and specifically disclaim any implied warranties or merchantability of
fitness for a particular purpose. While all attempts have been made to verify information, neither the author or the publisher nor the marketing agents assumes
any responsibility for errors, omissions, or contrary interpretation of the subject
matter whatever the circumstances. No warranty may be created or extended by
sales representatives or written sales materials. The advice and strategies contained herein may not be suitable for your situation. You should consult with a
professional where appropriate. Neither the publisher nor the author shall be li-
able for any loss of profit or any commercial damages, including but not limited
to special, incidental, consequential, or other damages.

For general information on our other products and services or for technical
support, please contact our technical support within the United States at pub@
innovative-publishers.com online at http://innovative-publishers.com.

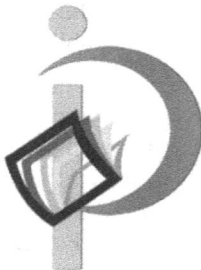

Innovative Publishers

Table of contents

Introduction to Weight Management

With the rapid rate at which obesity has spread over the last couple of decades, the importance of weight management programs has also grown as a consequence. Weight management program refers to all those activities that help an individual to either gain weight, lose weight or even to maintain it at the current level. In any of these goals, a weight management program targets increasing or maintaining the amount of lean muscle mass while decreasing the body fat percentage. Any other way of losing or gaining weight will be unhealthy in one aspect or another and may compromise health in the short term, but definitely in the long run.

Body Composition

Our body comprises of different components, namely fat, lean muscle, water, bones, organs etc. Each of them contributes to the total body weight. For each and every individual each of these constituent elements is present in different proportions. The ratio in which this distribution is present in any individual is called body composition. In the context of weight management, the division is done into two categories – fat mass and fat free mass. A healthy body composition is one in which the fat mass is low and fat free mass is higher. Through different weight management programs it is attempted to alter body composition in a manner that it boosts good health.

There are many techniques and methods to determine body composition. With technological advancements newer and more accurate equipments are available for performing body composition analysis. Traditional techniques such as skin fold measurements are easy to implement but have limited accuracy. Newer technologies such as ultrasound and bioelectric impedance analysis help in doing body composition analysis using simple and portable machines that give extremely accurate results as well. These different methods determine not only the amount of fat and lean muscle tissue but also provide a segmental analysis so that appropriate intervention strategies can be planned as part of the weight management program.

Doing body composition analysis on a regular basis should be included as part of any weight management strategy since it will help in monitoring the alterations taking place in the body as a result of the program. Since the body is undergoing change on a regular basis it is imperative that the program should also change accordingly. A program that was designed for the individual who weighed say 240 pounds will need to be changed when the person loses weight and weighs 200 pounds now. Body composition analysis also provides information on whether the weight loss is happening in a healthy manner or not. In case the weight loss happens at the expense of lean muscle or water then changes need to be done in the program so that these components can be restored to normal levels and fat loss targeted by introducing appropriate changes. A number of new age weight loss methods as well as gadgets are able to provide good results in terms of weight loss but they do it at the expense of good health. Doing a simple body composition analysis will reveal the true nature of these unhealthy methods and systems. Most new technologies also provide information on metabolic rate which is directly correlated the amount of lean mass in the body. Greater the lean mass higher will be the energy that is required by the body to maintain it. The measurement of metabolic rate helps in designing the exercise program as well as the calorie intake required as part of the diet & nutrition plan. Since the needs and requirement of each and every individual are different, the weight management strategy has to be necessarily different as well. Body composition analysis is the first step in designing a weight management program and should thereafter be done on a regular basis.

Problems with adverse body composition

A body composition analysis that reveals high fat percentage in comparison to lean muscle mass percentage points to obesity. Obesity is a modern day lifestyle disease that is essentially a silent killer. It indirectly leads to other physical as well as mental disorders, ailments and diseases that later on deplete the quality of life of the individual and in certain cases may even lead to death. The most common ailments that accompany obesity include type-2 diabetes, hypertension, cardiovascular & coronary artery disease, metabolic syndrome polycystic ovary syndrome and Dyslipidemia. Obesity also leads to gastrointestinal issues such as Cholelithiasis, GERD or Gastroesophageal Reflex Disease, Fatty Liver Disease, Colon Cancer and Hernia; genitourinary problems include erectile dysfunction, renal failure, incontinence and hypogonadism; Respiratory problems include sleep apnea, Hypoventilation syndrome and dyspnea. Apart from these physical ailments obesity also leads to psychological problems that arise from a diminished self confidence and if left unchecked may even lead to chronic depression.

Causes of Obesity

Obesity is caused by an energy intake in the form of diet that is not balanced by equivalent amount of physical activity. The basic law of conservation of energy cannot be violated at any cost and hence, energy excess will lead to weight gain while energy deficit will lead to weight loss. Energy input into the body is through the food that we eat. Energy output is the sum of a number of parameters that include – energy expended through physical exercise, energy spent in activities performed in daily life, basal metabolic rate or the energy required by the body to perform essential body functions such as respiration and digestion; in addition there are a few other parameters such as *thermic effect of food* and *adaptive thermogenesis* that add onto energy output but only in relatively small amounts. It is when the energy input becomes greater than energy output that the body starts storing this excess energy in the form of body fat. Some amount of fat is essential for efficient body functioning but when the fat percentage goes above certain levels it leads to obesity and consequently a host of other disorders and diseases.

This energy imbalance is the objective reason behind obesity but it is important to understand the underlying reasons why this imbalance is created. Imbalanced diet and sedentary lifestyle are the primary causes which get accentuated as a result of numerous personal, social, cultural and familial issues. Genetics and medical conditions also contribute towards increasing the fat mass in an individual. While most parameters seem to be alterable, some of these parameters may not seem to be in control of the individual and a situation of helplessness may be experienced. However, there are ways and means to counter any of these issues that gradually lead to weight loss in a healthy manner.

Genetic factors and Body Type

As mentioned above certain parameters that influence body composition cannot be modified. Genetic predisposition is one such parameter. Genetics define the body type of an individual which then affects the way in which the body reacts to a certain lifestyle and also to any alteration that is forced on this lifestyle. There are different classification techniques for differentiating between different body types.

1. The ancient Indian science of *Ayurveda* uses a classification method based on energy patterns or types. It is believed as per *Ayurveda* that the universe comprises of five basic elements – space, air, water, fire and earth. A combination of these basic elements is responsible for defining the human physiology. The basis of classification therefore is on the basis of energy patterns or *doshas* which comprise of one or more of these elements. The three *doshas* – *vata, pitta* and *kapha* define the person's physiology and all *Ayurvedic* treatments start from the identification of the *dosha* and identifying the imbalance in the *dosha* pattern. Once this is done remedial solution can be prescribed the aim of which is to restore the balance in the elements.

2. The second classification technique is based on the metabolic type. Under this classification technique the basis of differentiation between body types is the dominating gland in the endocrine system. It is believed that the biochemical reactions happening in the body of the individual are influenced and controlled by the dominating gland. This dominance of one particular gland over the others is built into the genetic structure and has a significant impact on the metabolic processes in the body. These metabolic processes take up raw materials such as carbohydrates, fats, proteins in different proportions and occur in the presence of catalysts that are available through micronutrients such as minerals and vitamins. The difference in proportions of raw material

utilized is due to the functioning differences between these glands of the endocrine system. The classification is done into 4 main categories – adrenal (controls reaction to environmental stresses and dangers), gonad (controls reproduction and growth), thyroid (controls metabolism) and pituitary (control the secretion of all glands) depending upon the dominating gland. Different diets and exercise routines are recommended for different body types.

3. The third classification technique and most commonly used in the context of weight management programs is on the basis of Somatotype. The system is based on identifying the association between psychological behavior patterns or temperament with the body structure of the individual. Under this system it is believed that the characteristic behavioral patterns as exhibited by an individual are typical of his or her own body type to a significantly large extent. The body type as in other classification systems is genetically predetermined. People having a similar body type are expected to show similar behavioral traits under this system. The system of classification is on the basis of the 3 elements or Somatotypes that are named after cell groups known as *germinal epithelium* formed during the growth of the embryo in the womb. The three Somatotypes are named after the three germ layers - *mesoderm, endoderm* and *ectoderm* and are therefore called Mesomorph, Endomorph and Ectomorph respectively. Mesomorphs are characterized by a predominance of lean muscle, connective tissues and bone; Endomorphs are characterized by a predominant roundness & softness in the different parts of the body as a consequence of excess body fat; Ectomorphs are characterized by fragility & linearity and are therefore possess frail and weak body structures which are devoid of fat as well as lean muscle. An individual may not necessarily be a pure Somatotype and can be a combination of one or more of these Somatotypes.

These body types are not inflexible to change arising from application of stimulus in the form of exercise and diet. Not each and every one possesses a dream body shape and structure by birth. Similarly, not everyone who has the nature predisposition to a good physique is able to maintain it. The genetic code embedded into our body in the form of body type plays a significant role in determining our body shape but it is not the only parameter. It is true that an Ectomorph may ingest large number of calories as part of diet and may perform rigorous strength training routines but still may find it difficult to add an extra pound of weight. Similarly, an endomorph may perform long duration cardiovascular workouts but still may not be able to shed those extra pounds of fat stored in the body. However, genetic predisposition only indicates the difficulty to create changes; nowhere does it mention that it is impossible. Moreover, in most cases an individual is a combination of Somatotypes which makes it possible to create changes in one direction or the other depending upon the requirement. It is therefore of utmost importance to identify the body type and the goals before designing an exercise program and diet plan. Once this identification has been done, adherence to a scientifically designed weight management program will lead to achievement of the desired targets that have been set.

Components of weight management program

A healthy weight management program should be based on the four pillars of wellness – physical fitness, balanced diet & nutrition, rest & relaxation and mental attitude. A balance between all the four components is crucial for the success of a weight management program. A good fitness routine which is not accompanied by an appropriate diet will not help the individual trying to lose weight. Similarly, a person who does not have the right mental frame of mind will find it extremely difficult to adhere to certain basic restrictions that such a program may impose; as a result of which the whole program fails. A weight management program needs to be customized according the needs and goals of the individual. This customization needs to be reflected in all the components as well. In case even one of them is not in sync it can derail the whole program itself.

Balanced diet & nutrition

A good balanced and nutritious diet is paramount to the success of a weight management program. Not only should it provide the right amount of energy depending upon the goals of the program, it should also provide the necessary micronutrients in adequate quantities for long term sustainable weight loss and overall health. A balanced diet incorporates energy compounds such as carbohydrates, fats and proteins, micronutrients such as vitamins and minerals as well as fiber and water in adequate quantities. As mentioned before the quantity and proportion of the main energy compounds depends on the goal of the program while micronutrients should be available to the body as per standard guidelines such as DV (Daily Value), RDA (Recommended Dietary Allowance) and EAR (Estimated Average Requirement).

In case the goal is to lose weight then an energy deficit needs to be created in a way that energy intake is less than energy output. This may involve reducing the quantities of the energy compounds from the normal diet and vice versa in case weight gain is the goal. As part of a weight management diet plan identifying the calorie content of meals is extremely crucial. To lose one pound of fat, a deficit of 3,500 calories needs to be created. This can be done by ensuring a regular deficit of 500 calories per day throughout the week. A gradual weight loss rate of one to two pounds per week is ideal for the body since it gets time to adapt to the changed conditions. Moreover, gradual weight loss ensures that there is least amount of muscle loss that happens as part of the weight loss process. This is where the efficacy of crash diets or very low calorie diets is questioned. Apart from loss of muscle tissue they cause micronutrient deficiency extremely dangerous to overall health. Certain research studies also confirm that such diets in fact may lead to fat gain since the body experiences starvation and tends to preserve the energy dense compounds for later utilization. This is done at the expense of lean muscle tissue which is difficult to maintain in the body.

In general any meal should include around 55 to 60% energy being provided through carbohydrates, 25 to 30% energy through fats and approximately 10 to 20% through proteins. This principally ensures that while all the energy requirements are met, nourishment of the body is not compromised upon. Even in case an energy deficit is required for losing weight it created in such a way that all nutrients including fats are available to the body for essential functions that need to be performed for healthy a mind & body.

Once the energy requirements have been calculated the next step in the preparation of a balanced diet plan is identification of the meals and meal content. By identification of the meals, it is intended to finalize the meal frequency and the meal timings such that they can be incorporated in the lifestyle in an easy manner. Too many alteration in the existing pattern of life make the adherence to the plan that much more difficult. Therefore, a diet plan should be designed taking into consideration the individual's lifestyle and preferences. In this context the question of meal frequency becomes a pertinent one. The three meal plan has been ingrained into modern day diets since it is conveniently adopted into work life pattern. It may not necessarily be as good and efficient for overall health as well as for weight loss in comparison to a high frequency diet plan such as a 6 meal plan.

Our body requires energy at a particular rate; this rate is defined by our metabolic rate but there may be spikes in demand such as the post exercise period. Clearly, the body does not require energy at the rate at which we eat and the rate at which the energy is released in our body upon digestion of food. In such a situation the excess energy needs to be stored in the body to be utilized at a later stage. The body can do it in the form of glycogen in the liver and muscles but once these limited space stores are filled up then it converts the extra energy into fat which can be stored all over the body. Secondly, whenever a heavy meal is consumed the insulin spike that occurs upon increase in glucose level in the blood, stays on for a longer period of time. In a similar manner this also results in storage of carbohydrates initially as glycogen but later on as fat. Smaller meals ensure that the body gets energy at a rate commensurate to its requirements so that it does not have to convert and store it as body fat. A high frequency 6 meal plan aids in this process of immediate utilization.

The other factor is the proportion of energy that is derived from stored energy reserves versus that derived from food that has been consume in the recent past. The body stores energy compounds like glucose in the blood, glycogen or long chain glucose molecules in the liver and muscles. And fat in the adipose tissue. Whenever the requirement for energy arises the body meets it through one of these sources. When extra carbohydrates are ingested as part of the meal the body stops utilizing the fat stored in the body, on top of this, the extra carbohydrate gets converted into fat. In a high frequency meal plan, the amount of carbohydrates consumed in any meal is limited, which prevents prolonged insulin spike from occurring. This helps in preventing conversion of carbohydrates into fat and also helps in utilizing stored fat for meeting energy requirement.

As part of weight management programs high frequency smaller meals are often suggested due to the aforementioned reasons. The other psychological advantages offered by these plans are beneficial in ensuring adherence during the initial difficult periods of change. By trimming down meal quantities and increasing frequency, cravings that lead to unplanned eating can be prevented. Since, as part of the meal itself there are many meals, the meal content is pre-planned and hence, the chances of eating something unhealthy out of the diet plan are reduce. Uncontrolled hunger pangs are also not experienced since the gap between meals is shorter. This has a dual advantage – apart from preventing binge eating it also helps in avoiding overeating during the main meals. The effect of frequent meals on metabolism has also been seen to be positive in nature. By eating frequent meals, the body is not allowed to go onto starvation mode and thereby the metabolism is maintained at a high since there it is made to experience a near constant availability of food and energy. Increased metabolism helps in burning the extra fat reserves in the body and hence helps in losing weight in a desirable manner. In summary, a high frequency smaller meal plan seems to be much more effective in reducing body fat percentage in comparison to the modern day three meal plan. This loss in fat percentage is ideal for weight loss as well as weight gain. Hence such a meal plan can be made an integral part of any weight management program.

Physical exercise as part of weight management plan

The second pillar in a healthy weight management program is regular physical exercise at the right intensity. It helps in increasing the energy output to create the deficit that is essential for weight loss to take place. In case weight gain is the goal, exercise provides stimulus forcing the body to grow to meet the additional demands placed on it. Whatever the goals may be, like a healthy weight management plan, a healthy exercise routine should include all the components – cardiovascular endurance, muscular endurance, muscular strength and flexibility.

1. Cardiovascular endurance exercises include all those exercises that involve repetitive movement of large muscle groups at a heart rate greater than resting heart rate. Exercises include running, jogging, swimming, cycling, rowing etc. The role of the cardiovascular system is to ensure efficient delivery of oxygen to different parts of the body. Performing regular cardio exercises not only improves the delivery mechanism of oxygen but also helps improve the efficiency of the vascular system and the exercising muscles to take up and utilize the oxygen delivered. Chronic adaptations as a result of cardio activities help in preventing cardiovascular and coronary artery diseases, metabolic disorders such as diabetes and metabolic syndrome and may also help in preventing certain forms of cancer.

2. Muscular endurance exercises help improve the endurance of different muscle groups in the body. Numerous activities of daily life involve repeated movements to be performed of a particular type and therefore utilize a particular muscle group. Improved muscular endurance helps in performing these movements without experiencing too much fatigue in the exercising muscle.

3. Muscular strength is the ability of a particular muscle to lift heavy loads. In daily life, the requirement to lift and carry heavy load often arises but infrequently. If the body is deconditioned to perform such a movement then there is risk of injury. Strength training exercises help in increasing lean muscle tissue in the body as well as improves the quality of

bone health by strengthening them. In such a manner it helps in performing activities of daily life.

4. Flexibility refers to pain free range of motion around a joint. This is one of the most neglected aspects of fitness and as age progresses it becomes the most important component. Flexibility training in the form of static stretches held for moderate to long durations helps in improving flexibility which then reduced the risk of injuries.

All these components of exercise are important in the context of weight management but more emphasis is directed towards exercises such as cardiovascular workouts. These exercises increase the heart rate in such a manner that the extra demands placed on the body force it to rely on stored energy reserves in the body. By careful planning of diet and intensity of workout it is possible to selectively utilize fat stored in the body for meeting the energy requirements. A balanced routine should include 40 minutes of moderate intensity aerobic activity for 3 to 4 times a week, strength training or resistance training of all the muscle groups at least twice a week and static stretching to improve flexibility should also be incorporated at least 2 to 3 times a week. Such a balanced workout leads to weight loss as well as improves overall physical fitness.

Rest & Relaxation

It is important to understand that the actual growth and development of the body does not take place while exercise is being performed. Exercise only provides the stimulus required for growth and development of tissues. The other ingredients that ensure that the purpose is fulfilled are balanced & nutritious diet and rest & relaxation. Post exercise when the body rests and is provided energy and nutrition is the time when the actual growth happens. At this stage the energy requirements should be met from within the fat stores for weight loss to take place. In case this is not done, the body will strip lean muscle tissue to meet the demands post by exercise. Also, in case enough rest is not provided to the body, the chance of overtraining leading to injury increases manifold. Adequate amount of rest and relaxation also helps in maintaining hormonal balance in the body. This is also crucial for healthy weight management.

Mental attitude

A perfectly designed diet plan or a perfectly designed exercise routine is of no use if the individual for whom it is designed is not able to adhere to it. This is where the role of a positive mental attitude comes into picture. Psychological factors play an important role in weight management than is generally imagined. In fact adherence to any plan is solely dependent on the attitude a person carries towards the lifestyle alteration that is being imposed as part of the plan. In case the weight management program is looked at as a set of limitations or restrictions that is forced, the chances of adherence in the short run as well as over a period of time diminish significantly. On the contrary an individual adopting a positive attitude looks at the program as a new positive lifestyle which is embraced with vigour and excitement.

Yoga for weight management

'Yoga' is derived from '*yuj*' in Sanskrit which means 'to unite'. Originating in ancient India, it is a unique combination of mental, physical as well as spiritual disciplines. This union that yoga refers to is the union of the individual with the universal. Yoga is believed to have originated more than 25,000 years ago and contrary to common knowledge it is not just a sequence of poses and postures for improving health and fitness. It is an ancient science that includes tools such as *pranayama* or breathing methods and techniques, meditation also called *dhyana* and finally physical postures or *asanas*.

The modern form of yoga is believed to have begun with Parliament of Religions convened in Chicago in the year 1893. In the convention *Swami Vivekanand* had a deep impact on the thinking of the audience. In subsequent tours in the United States he promoted various aspects of yoga. These talks and lectures led to yoga shedding the tag of a purely religious practice and being accepted by the western world. In the years since then health benefits emanating through regular yogic practices have been researched, documented and published all over the world. It is estimated that in the US alone more than 25 million people practice yoga on a regular basis.

The myriad benefits of yoga include physiological benefits such as improved flexibility, increased strength, better posture, weight loss, effective breathing, stronger immune system, improved bone strength and improvement in medical conditions such as migraine and insomnia; psychological benefits include stress relief, greater awareness, improved energy levels and an overall feeling of inner peace. Yoga is quite efficient in weight loss as well. It advocates a multi dimensional approach that incorporates physical, emotional and spiritual components and does not superficially work on eliminating the symptoms alone. The root cause of the problem is targeted through yoga to deal with the weight problem. It therefore involves detoxification, increasing metabolism, achieving hormonal balance, improving observation & awareness and cardiovascular endurance. Certain forms of yoga prescribe movements done at a rapid pace in a sequential manner that elevates heart rate to moderate or high levels and in such a manner mimic cardiovascular activities. This is very similar to circuit training which is a form of strength training where each muscle group is exercises one after the other without any rest. Such workout principles help in weight loss since heart rate is maintained at a moderate to high level for considerable duration. Apart from the *asanas* that are practiced, *kriyas* such as *kapalbhati* done at a vigorous intensity provides a good cardiovascular endurance workout. Different *asanas* also have different effects on the mind as well. Certain movements performed at a particular pace are known to provide calmness, while other movements help in boosting energy levels. Yoga *asanas* also improve thyroid and pituitary health and balanced secretion of hormones helps in improving metabolism to suit the body's requirements. Other benefits such as reduction in anxiety and detoxification of the body indirectly help in losing weight in a healthy manner. The psychological benefits such as improved awareness and sense of calmness help in immensely improving adherence to weight management program since they bring about a positive attitude towards the entire process.

Meditation for weight management

Meditation refers to the process of reflection and contemplation that helps in calming the mind and in this way relieves stress and anxiety. It has been commonly linked with religion and prayer across many cultures since ancient times. It is often thought of as a tool to improve concentration and as an aid to attaining peace of mind, a path to God and spirituality. Meditation is commonly done by mental exercises that include concentrated breathing, single point focussing as well as chanting. In some cultures it is performed by being completely detached from external worldly contacts while in others the person may interact with the outside world while practicing meditation.

Meditation has developed over centuries and across cultures and civilizations. There is no one form of meditation that fits all the requirements and is ideal for each and everyone practicing it. Which form suits whom depend on factors like state of mind, personality traits and external surroundings. The meditation form that should be practiced is the one in which the person feels most comfortable rather than going after something which is perceived by people in close contact to be most helpful. There is no one single source or authority or text that is referred to for meditation practices. Numerous different forms have evolved over ages each having certain distinct characteristics. A high proportion of these forms though, involve awareness of breath as the underlying platform on which meditation is practiced. Different types of meditation include the following:

1. *Mindfulness meditation* is a popular practice in the West in which awareness of the surroundings is not blocked out. The idea in this practice is to allow all the thoughts to flow into the mind without focusing on any single one of them. This form does not necessarily require quiet and peaceful surroundings and can be performed anywhere. Breathing like most meditation forms is important but is not the primary and sole element. It is a form which is suited to beginners who may find concentrating and blocking out thoughts to focus on nothingness extremely difficult.

2. *Focused meditation* involves focusing on a single thought throughout the practice session. The point of focus can be internal like an imagined object and can also be external in nature like a chant. The emphasis is not on the thought but

on the process of maintaining concentration and not losing focus.

3. *Spiritual meditation* is a form which is closely interlinked with religion and is suited to individuals who offer prayers as part of their daily rituals. The emphasis is on communication and interaction with God and union with the Universal.

4. *Trance based meditation* is an advanced form of spiritual meditation that involves reaching a state of trance by losing self control induced by usage of intoxicating substances. Since the person practicing this form of meditation may not have any memory of the experience, it has a very limited usage, if any, on daily life.

5. *Movement meditation* is a form in which the practice involves constant movement. These movements can be slow & rhythmic in nature such as swaying of the body. These gentle movements are believed to have a calming influence on the mind.

6. *Other forms of meditation* include mantra meditation, transcendental meditation, *kundalini* meditation, *Qi gong* meditation and *Zazen* meditation. Each of them originating in different ages and different parts of the world; differing in the way they are practiced and in terms of their end objectives as well.

Since it is not an exact science, the benefits of meditation cannot be directly and objectively measured. Interest in the scientific community has increased immensely as a result of observations, but studies and research has not determined conclusive proof of benefits derived from meditation. Physical benefits include elimination of stress leading to improvement in conditions such as hypertension and diabetes. The vibrations released are also known to have the added effect of diminishing the negative impact of the disease. Meditation is known to reduce the level of Cortisol and hence reduces stress levels; it also reduces the accumulation of lactic acid which is associated with anxiety. Meditation helps in breath control thereby reducing heart rate and helping the body fight against hypertension; it helps to improve immunity, provides balance to the hormonal system, improves fertility, reduces cholesterol level and helps in weight loss.

While weight loss cannot be directly achieved through meditation it has a more important role to play than any other parameter including physical exercise and diet & nutrition. Meditation does not burn fat in the body but it provides a frame of mind and attitude that is crucial for the efficient functioning of the tools that result in weight loss. Without a positive frame of mind adherence to the weight management program is practically impossible. Meditation helps in identifying the root cause of the weight problem and it does not superficially work on the symptoms of the problem. Even if an individual on a weight loss program is able to achieve weight loss, it may not be sustainable and permanent in case the root cause is not tackled. Meditation helps in improving self control and thereby increases determination that helps in adhering to the program. Moreover, the positive attitude with which the program is adopted magnifies the benefits that may be derived. From the psychological perspective of filling in voids, people have a tendency to go on binges – commonly termed as emotional eating. Meditation helps by working on elimination of desire itself helping the individual practicing it to remain unaffected by the pressures of daily home and work life. The positive attitude that is manifested helps to attain a balance in life. This balance prevents excessive emotions either positive or negative. The person thus practicing experiences an ever prevalent calmness irrespective of the external environment and the alterations that these parameters may undergo. While meditation objectively may not lead to weight loss in the conventional sense, it empowers the individual with a positive attitude – the most useful tool in attaining any weight loss goal.

Meditation also provides numerous psychological benefits. It helps ease stress & anxiety as mentioned earlier. A person becomes calm & composed and is able to visualize the external world with detachment helping in decision making process. Meditation also recharges and provides a feeling of rejuvenation which increases efficiency of all work that the person indulges in. Practicing meditation on a regular basis provides greater mental control that helps in curbing fluctuations in mood and emotion. The spiritual benefits that are derived from regular practice of meditation are manifested in the attitude of kindness and compassion towards others. Union of mind, body and soul leads to an infinite source of love. All these benefits from meditation practice helps produce a balanced personality unfazed by external events and conditions.

Conclusion

For a successful weight management program it is imperative that all these components or pillars be incorporated. When these pillars are not in sync the chances of success of these plans reduces considerably. In fact, neglecting any one of these components may compromise short term as well as long term health and wellness. On the other hand when the wavelengths of the efforts do not match it is very unlikely that the weight management goals are achieved. A positive attitude towards a weight management program that includes a well rounded physical fitness routine, a balanced diet & nutrition plan and sufficient rest & relaxation is almost a guarantee to achieving long term and sustainable weight loss.

Yoga

What is yoga?

'Yoga', derived from the Sanskrit word *'yuj'* literally meaning 'to unite', is a combination of physical, mental and spiritual disciplines finding its origin in ancient India. The union referred to in the name is that of the individual with the universal spirit. It is one of the most ancient sciences and its origin is dated back to the origin of civilization itself. According to Hindu mythology, it is believed to have originated some 26,000 years ago in the age referred to as *Satyug* or the golden age; an age with an everlasting abundance of peace with people living harmoniously in their quest for the eternal truth. A few classical texts in fact propound *Lord Shiva*, the Hindu God as the first yogic teacher whereas the *Bhagwad Gita,* the holy Hindu scripture advocates *Lord Krishna* as the first teacher. The primary tools commonly used to practice yoga include physical postures or *asanas*, breathing techniques or *pranayama* and meditation or *dhyana.*

Yoga is a practical science or a discipline which is put to use to attain a specific goal. The purpose of yoga in general, is linked to the theological or philosophical school it is associated with. In some schools the purpose is devotion to take pleasure from constant experience of God, while in others it is the experience of *Brahman* or that which pervades all things. In modern times though, yoga is commonly understood as being a combination of numerous physical postures and breathing techniques that helps in elimination of various health problems and ailments, at the same time providing relaxation by alleviating stress.

We might know a bit about yoga, but to understand it in a better manner, it is important to understand the history of yoga right from the time of its origin.

Origin and history of yoga

Until recently it was believed by numerous western scholars that yoga originated around 500 BC, which is roughly the time of the Buddha, founder of Buddhism. In the 1920's, archaeologists discovered the Indus valley civilization. In the excavated material were several seals that depicted common yoga and meditation poses.

These seals were dated to the third millennium BC. Despite the absence of concrete proof, there is a certain resemblance between the postures depicted in these excavated seals and yoga practices of a later date. The history of yoga can be classified into four categories:

Vedic Yoga

Vedas are the oldest scriptures in the world. They were composed in a very archaic version of Sanskrit and were passed on from one generation to the next only by word of mouth. Considering the massive size of the scriptures such a process seems simply unfathomable, yet it is true beyond doubt. The *Vedas* mean knowledge and were essentially a collection of hymns. The four Vedas included *rig veda (rig* meaning praise) – the foremost scripture which has references that suggest that certain components may have been composed as long ago as the third millennium BC. The other three Vedas are *yajur veda, sama veda* and *atharva veda* essentially books of songs, rituals and spells respectively. The people during this age relied upon vedic seers or *rishis* to teach them the essence of life and the concepts of divine harmony. These seers lived in seclusion in forests and were known to possess powers of intuition gained through spiritual practice. The yoga of this period was connected to ritual life. By performing specific rituals with extreme focus levels it was aimed to enjoin the material and spiritual world. Such strong focus over prolonged periods for overcoming the limitations of the mind is the essence of vedic yoga.

Pre–classical Yoga

The pre–classical period covers a period of over 2,000 years, right until 200 AD. The yoga of this period is characterized by the Upanishads which is where the first usage of the term yoga seems to appear. There are more than 200 scriptures as part of the Upanishads which contain the essence of Vedas – ultimate unity of the entire universe is the hidden teaching. *Katha Upanishads* define yoga as the achievement of the supreme state through cessation of all mental activities. This is done through a gradual control gained over all the senses. Concepts such as *kundalini* and *chakra* (explained later) as well as the relationship between breath and thought process are mentioned in these texts. However, the goal of yoga in the Upanishads was clearly the transcendent self.

The *Bhagwad Gita* was the song of the Lord as narrated by Lord Krishna to the warrior prince Arjun. The usage of the term yoga has been done in numerous ways within the text. Apart from the traditional practice & meditation it contains information on *karma yoga* or action, *bhakti yoga* or devotion, *jnana yoga* or knowledge.

The *Mahabharata* and *Ramayana* are two of the greatest Indian epics – *Mahabharata* being the longest poem in the world (more than six times the content of Odyssey and Iliad combined). These epics contain the teachings of many schools of the era which taught the practice of deep meditation. Yogis practicing these techniques could transcend mind & body thus understanding their true spiritual essence and the unity of the one and all.

Classical Yoga

This period between 500 BC to 500 AD was the period of Mauryan and Gupta dynasties. It is during this period that different forms of yoga began to emerge in different Hindu, Buddhist and Jain philosophical schools. Classical yoga is marked by the creation of *Yoga Sutra*. It was created by Patanjali and is considered the culmination of the systematization process of yoga that had started at the beginning of this period. They were written around 200 AD and seem to have considerable influence from previous schools of the era. The Yoga Sutras are terse as well as complicated. They are often studied along with *Yoga Bhashya* which is essentially a collection of commentaries on *Yoga Sutra* written in the fifth century providing explanations to cryptic and complicated components. The form of yoga arising from *yoga sutras* is called *Raja yoga* and it emphasizes control over the mind.

The *Yoga Sutra* contains 196 *sutras* or threads divided into chapters:

1. *Samadhi Pada* which deals with the nature of *Samadhi* or perfect concentration

2. *Sadhana Pada* deals with the process of refining and cleansing the mind, body & soul

3. *Vibhuti Pada* deals with yogic properties and integration achieved through meditation. It also deals with super natural powers and gifts.

4. *Kaivalya Pada* deals in the relationship of the yogi with the soul

The *Yoga Sutras* lead to the birth of the system known as *Ashtanga Yoga* or eight–limbed form of yoga. It is the core characteristic of every form of *Raja yoga* being practiced today. The eight components are as following:

1. *Yama* means social restraints and covers the 5 abstentions – *ahimsa* or non–violence, *asteya* or non–covetousness, *brahmacharya* or celibacy, *satya* or truth and finally *aparigraha* or non–possessiveness

2. *Niyama* means observing purity & tolerance and covers the 5 observances – *shaucha* or purity, *tapas* or austerity, *santosha* or satisfaction, *svadhyaya* or study of the scriptures to understand God and finally *ishvara–pranidhana* or surrender to the almighty

3. *Asana* means seat, referring to the position for meditation but covers all the postures and physical exercises

4. *Pranayama* means breath regulation and control

5. *Pratyahara* means withdrawal of senses while preparing for meditation

6. *Dharana* means concentration and focusing attention on one specific object

7. *Dhyana* means meditation

8. *Samadhi* means ecstasy through liberation

It was believed as part of this school that individual is composed of both matter and spirit. Contrary to Vedic and pre–classical yoga, it was believed that it was essential to separate the two for attaining purity of spirit.

Post–classical Yoga

This is the post–Patanjali period up till present date during which numerous schools have sprung up that are derived from or in some cases even independent from his work. During this period, the focus shifted to the present, and emphasis was on accepting reality and living in the present moment rather than focusing only on liberation. There was a distinct turn in attention from purely the mind & soul to the physical body. Yogis in previous eras concentrated upon the union with the universal one, however now, attention towards the body was given equal emphasis. This resulted in development of practices that rejuvenated the body in a way to promote and prolong a healthy life.

Bhakti yoga became popular as part of the *bhakti movement* in the 12th century AD. It advocated meditative practices with devotion towards God. Yogis such as *Surdasa, Meerabai* and *Tulsidasa* popularized *bhakti yoga. Hatha yoga* period started from the 9th century AD and was at its peak during the 14th century AD. It was started by *Gorakshanath* and *Matsyendranath* who were *shivaite* ascetics. It is sometimes also called psychophysical yoga because of its basis on the premise that a pure physical body will lead to a pure mind. It takes up the *asanas* from *yoga sutras* and converts them into full postures; it is these postures that are associated with yoga today. Many texts have been written during this period and different personalities came to the forefront with their schools of teaching. A few prominent ones include *Sri Shankaracharya* in the 8th century AD and *Ramanujacharya* in the 11th century AD.

Modern yoga

Modern yoga is considered to begin with the Parliament of Religions that was convened in the year 1893 in Chicago. In this convention *Swami Vivekanand* created a lasting impression in the minds of the audience. He was the first person to disseminate and promote various aspects of yoga to the western world during his tours to the US and Europe. In continuation with the gradual introduction of physical aspects of yoga in the previous era, modern yoga is also associated with *asanas* as a form of exercise. Gradually yoga has been able to shed its connection with purely religious contexts, making it generally more acceptable to world audience. Over the years, the health benefits from regular practice of yoga has been documented and published widely. As a result of which more 20 million people practice yoga in the US alone.

Different types of yoga

Since the classical period numerous forms of yoga have been taught by various schools. Each of them has different driving philosophies as well as distinct methods of practice.

1. *Raja yoga* – It refers to the system advocated by Patanjali in *Yoga Sutra*. The eight limb system described in the previous section forms the basis of *raja yoga*. It is a form which is practiced by refinement of behavior through restraint, discipline, physical health through postures, breathing techniques, sensory withdrawal, concentration, meditation and finally liberation.

2. *Hatha yoga* – *Hatha yoga* is based on the book called *Hatha yoga pradipika* written around the 12th century AD by *Swami Swatmarama*. It is a systematic combination of techniques aimed at cleansing of mind & body and effects consciousness. It is a combination of *asanas* or practice of full body postures, *pranayama* or breathing techniques, *mudras* or gestures signifying mental attitudes, *bandhas* or energy locks, *nada* or sound and meditation. It is one of the most commonly practiced forms of yoga and is generally associated as representative of yoga for most people. It is believed that if practiced in the right manner it not only helps in getting rid of various mental and physical ailments but also increases the *pranic energy* leading to stability, sound health as well as lightness of body & mind.

3. *Mantra yoga* – *Mantras* are essentially verses from the Vedas. This school of yoga believed that the chanting of these *mantras* will lead to salvation or union with the one. The bottom line though is that one needs to have complete and unconditional faith in the power of the *mantra* without which it will simply be recitation, which will simply be futile. *Mantras* are generally classified into 2 categories – *tantric* (originated

from the *tantras* and practiced for certain specific purposes) and *puranic* (relatively simple form that can be easily learnt and practiced). The selection of the *mantra* or verse can be done by the Guru (also called *guru mantra*), it could be the *universal mantra or Om,* it could even be based on the basic inherent nature of the individual (different mantras such as *gayatri mantra* and *mahamrutyunjay mantra* suit different natures of individuals)

4. *Bhakti yoga – Bhakti* or complete devotion to God is the basis of this form of yoga. The concept of personal God also came into picture during the *bhakti movement*. The universal supreme is manifested in various forms, be it Krishna, Rama, Buddha or Jesus. This form of yoga works by the process of channelizing the emotional energy towards the object of devotion. Suppressed emotions in the individual are considered to be the reason behind all forms of physical as well as mental ailments, through *bhakti yoga* these suppressed emotions get released leading to purification of mind & body.

5. *Karma yoga – Karma* literally means work in Sanskrit and this form of yoga emphasizes complete devotion to work as the path to salvation. Whenever a person does some work there is an outcome or an end to which the person starts getting attached to. In the practice of *karma yoga* this attachment is what one aims to cut out so that selfless work is what remains. In this state the mind becomes stable and is not affected by the ups & downs that are associated with the output of what work one does. In this state of mind work comes to represent devotion and it should therefore be practiced without attachment of any kind to the end result.

6. *Jnana yoga* –In Sanskrit *Jnana* literally means knowledge, but in the current context it means wisdom attained through self awareness. Through a process of meditation it is possible to attain wisdom and understand true nature of inner knowledge. Self realization is the goal that is sought through meditation.

7. *Kundalini yoga* – There are psychic *chakras* that are believed

to exist in each and every individual. The 6 main chakras include *mooladhara* or coccygeal, *swadishtana* or sacral, *manipura* or solar, *anahata* or cardiac, *vishuddhi* or cervical, *ajna* or pineal, *bindu and sahasrara* or cerebellum. Through the practice of this form of yoga the goal is to awaken these various *chakras* or psychic centers. There are different layers of the mind, each associated with a particular level of consciousness and different *chakras*. Through *kundalini yoga* a yogi tries to awaken the higher level *chakras* through deep concentration that then forces their arousal. The awakening can be stimulated by a combination of *asanas, pranayama, mudras and bandhas*. Even other forms of yoga such as *mantra yoga* can be utilized to cause the awakening.

8. *Swara yoga* – *Swara* in Sanskrit means note or sound. It also represents the flow of air through the nostrils. Thus this form of yoga aims at union through the manipulation and control of breath. Whereas *pranayama* relates only to the ways in which breath can be controlled and is basically a group of breathing techniques, *swara yoga* also incorporates observation and study of breath apart from manipulation and control. Therefore it more comprehensive in nature.

Apart from these, there have been numerous schools that have sprung up of late, specifically in the 19th and 20th century AD. Quite a few of them have gained popularity in the west. These schools have been able to translate complicated ritualistic forms of yoga to simpler forms which can be practiced by a layman. By their emphasis on the health benefits derived from regular practice of yoga these schools have been able to engage the attention of the masses by their emphasis on present world real life. A few forms that have gained quite a bit of prominence of late include the following:

1. *Anusara yoga* is one of the relatively newer forms of yoga started in 1997, which is a combination of difficult postures but emphasizes the playful spirit and opening up of the heart while still performing the *asanas* with correct alignment.

2. *Bikram Yoga* was started by Bikram Choudhury and is based

on the belief of a comprehensive workout that includes muscular strength, cardiovascular endurance, muscular endurance and flexibility. Unique about this form of yoga is that it is practiced in a heated environment usually at 95 to 105 degrees Fahrenheit. It is believed that in such an environment yoga promotes detoxification.

3. *Iyengar Yoga* is one of the most popular forms of yoga and was developed by B.K.S.Iyengar in the 1970's. It is a form of *hatha yoga* that uses different types of props such as cushions, blocks and belts that helps even the elderly and disabled to perform the *asanas.* These *asanas* are generally held for longer periods of time, a minute or so or may be even more. The slow movements along with usage of props that enable everyone to participate have made this form of yoga extremely popular.

4. *Power Yoga* is the modern version of *ashtanga yoga,* an American interpretation that includes most of the *asanas* being performed with vigor. The *asanas* resemble callisthenic workouts such as toe touches, push-ups and head stands. It lays emphasis on moving from one *asana* to another without any rest. Such fast paced continuous aerobic activity leads to burning fat and consequently healthy weight loss.

These newer forms of yoga have adapted themselves in a manner to appeal to the masses and make yoga accessible to everyone. Maintaining the basic premises of traditional yoga forms, these new schools add variety in a manner that they provide a holistic workout to the person practicing yoga. Gradually emphasis has shifted from yoga being a spiritual study to it becoming a practice for achieving and maintaining a healthy body and a calm and peaceful mind.

Benefits of Yoga

It is commonly believed that practicing yoga on a regular basis increases flexibility and promotes balance and coordination. However, this is a myopic viewpoint because most people understand yoga as a combination of *asanas* or body postures. Yoga practiced in its entirety not only has physiological benefits but also has a tremendous positive impact on the psychological and spiritual fronts of life.

Physiological benefits

1. Flexibility – The various *asanas* or postures help in stretching various muscles of the body. These postures are very similar to static stretches that are performed slowly and in which position is held for a brief period of time. Often people feel they are too stiff or old to perform yoga; on the contrary yoga is for everyone. Slow, controlled movements ensure that the chances of any kind of injury diminish considerably. At the same time within a short duration of practice benefits begin to be visible. Even an extremely unfit individual who is not able to flex a particular muscle about a joint is able to see improvements with a couple of weeks itself. Whenever we utilize our muscles for some activity of daily life or for even exercise, there is a build up in the short term and some amount of residual accumulation in the long run of lactic acid, a waste product of anaerobic activity. This leads to stiffness, exhaustion, fatigue and pain. Through regular practice of yoga *asanas* dispersion of this lactic acid takes place.

    Apart from the muscles in the body there are numerous other connective tissues such as ligaments and tendons. These tissues basically connect muscles and bones and also help control unwarranted movement of a joint above an acceptable range of motion. Athletes performing strenuous physical exercise and activities as well as general population are susceptible to injuries of these soft connective tissues. Yoga helps in increasing the mobility and flexibility of these tissues too and helps in preventing injuries. Improvement in range of motion about a joint and overall flexibility is by far the most commonly accepted reason as to why people start practicing yoga on a regular basis.

2. Strength – While practicing yoga, one is required to hold the various *asanas* or postures which required continuous recruitment of muscle fibers of various muscle groups. Nu-

merous of these postures require load bearing of body weight which requires muscle contraction to take place. Simultaneously, to maintain balance in these postures neuro-muscular coordination is required and that also recruits different muscle fibers. Overall strengthening of upper body, lower body and core takes place. This includes strengthening of not only major muscle groups such as shoulders, arms, hamstrings, quadriceps and abdominal group but also of smaller muscles of the back and neck, which prevent occurrences of common chronic ailments such as back pain and neck pain.

3. Posture – With increased flexibility and muscular strength, posture also improves. Almost all the standing as well as sitting exercises recruit and consequently strengthen the core muscles since they help in maintaining the poses for longer periods of time. As a result of this posture improves drastically, and a person is able to sit, stand and walk in the correct posture. An increased level of awareness helps in correcting any slouch or slump. Most chronic muscular pains of the neck and back are a direct consequence of an inappropriate posture. By working on the source of the problem, yoga helps in eliminating these issues.

4. Weight loss – One of the most sought after benefits that pulls people towards yoga is weight loss. Yoga works on both sides of the problem, helps in reducing weight as well as works in reducing the tendency to gain weight. By working on physical aspects fat burning takes place during and after a yoga session. At the same time, by working on the mental aspects one is able to concentrate and adhere to weight loss plans by eating, thinking and resting healthy. Many forms of yoga involve fast, continuous and vigorous movement that helps to burn calories and thereby account for weight loss. We shall look at this aspect in detail in a subsequent section.

5. Breathing – A predominant component of yoga is *pranayama* or the set of breathing exercises that are performed. Deep and concentrated breathing helps improve lung capacity as well as respiratory rate. This is of immense importance dur-

ing sports and endurance activities. A number of elite sports athletes nowadays are turning to yogic practices to improve their endurance and consequently athletic performance.

6. Cardiovascular endurance – 'Cardio' means heart and 'Vascular' means blood vessels. Together, 'Cardiovascular' system refers to the system in the body which provides oxygen to different parts of the body and helps utilize this oxygen to perform work. This includes involuntary activities such as beating of the heart controlled by the myocardial muscles as well as voluntary activities such as lifting a weight. All these activities require oxygen and the cardiovascular system is responsible for providing this efficiently. Yoga *asanas* help in lowering blood pressure levels and is immensely helpful in people having hypertension. It also helps in lowering the heart rate. Numerous studies have been conducted in this field, specially aiming to prove the positive effects of yoga on the cardiovascular system. Most of these studies provide a direct positive correlation. Apart from this, there is significant evidence that yoga helps in lowering cholesterol and triglyceride levels in the blood. Certain forms of yoga such as power yoga involve fast, continuous movement through various *asanas* and are extremely useful in cardiovascular conditioning.

7. Improved immunity – Regular practice of yoga has also been seen to increase antioxidant levels resulting in improved immunity. Not only does this mean lesser susceptibility to illness but also a lower chance of getting these ailments and diseases in the first place, all because of a better immune system protecting the body.

8. Helps in injury rehabilitation – Forms of yoga such as *Iyengar yoga* involve slow and controlled movements. Postures are held in position for a brief while but for much longer a duration than normal. It is therefore easily performed by people beginning practice of yoga as well old people who are relatively unfit. Simultaneously, it is equally helpful for people who are recovering from injuries, specifically mus-

culoskeletal injuries such as muscle pulls and repetitive stress injuries. Slow movements ensure that chances of injury are low and a person performs these *asanas* to the extent to which he or she is comfortable. The usage of props such as blocks, belts, blankets etc. make it easier for an individual to move closer to the perfect posture. Gradually the range of motion about joints increases as the injured soft tissues heal and become more and more flexible.

9. Improved bone mineral density – A number of yoga *asanas* are body weight bearing exercises. Our bones follow a rule, 'form follows function' which means that the more stress (under a particular range) that they undergo, the stronger they become. In such a manner yoga helps in increasing the bone mineral density. Post menopause women are susceptible to considerable loss of bone mineral and osteoporosis. Yoga helps prevent this loss of bone density.

10. Effects on medical conditions

   a. Migraine & headaches – Through an improved blood circulation and consequently better oxygen delivery to the brain, yoga helps in reducing and sometimes even eliminating the occurrences of headaches and migraines

   a. Insomnia – People practicing yoga on a regular basis experience better, deeper and a more relaxed sleep. Problems such as insomnia are eliminates due to physiological benefits of yoga as well as psychological ones which lead to lower amounts of stress experienced

   a. Treatment of cancer – Yoga is being increasingly used for treatment of cancer. It helps to decrease anxiety, pain and depression. Studies have found evidence that yoga leads to significantly lesser stress and mood disturbances as a result of which it is being used in cancer treatment

   a. Yoga is also used in the treatment of schizophrenia where reduced stress and improved cognitive behavior lead to lower chances of relapse and better overall quality of life. Other chronic ailments for which yoga is used as a part of a comprehensive treatment plan include asthma, multiple sclerosis and arthritis

Psychological benefits

1. Stress relief – Regular practice of yoga helps in getting stress levels down considerably. Even a regular 10 minute routine on a daily basis has shown to provide positive results. Yoga *asanas, pranayama* and meditation all help in relieving stress. In fact, yoga is incorporated as part of psychological therapy for treatment of stress related issues such as anxiety disorder and clinical depression.

2. Inner peace – Yoga helps in experiencing the inner peace within. A person does not have to depend on a vacation to go to a place that is away from the hustle & bustle of daily life. By practicing yoga one becomes aware of the immense peace that can be found within oneself. It is by far one of the best ways to calm a disturbed mind. It is in fact quite commonly used in helping people who have undergone some traumatic experience.

3. Greater awareness and observation – Due to the constant stresses of daily life, both at work and at home, one forgets to live in the present. Life is then dictated by what happens in the past and all our decisions are based on our self created image of the future. Yoga helps in understanding this very basic tendency of the mind. Through meditation it helps us in increasing our awareness and observation and helps us come back to the present. It helps us stay happy in the awareness of *what is* rather than worrying about *what can be.*

4. Increased energy levels – Even a short duration yoga session of only ten minutes helps one unwind. During the day when one feels energy sapped, yoga can help rejuvenate and reenergize within a few minutes. It thus gives us a feeling of renewed energy and acts like a energy booster in this regard

5. Better intuition – It has been experienced that yoga through

its meditative component helps improve intuition. Belief in positive results helps us realize what is best and what needs to be done – our intuitive capabilities improve. It is not something that can be researched and scientifically proven in a laboratory. It needs to be believed in and experienced.

Concept of Weight Management

Before we discuss how yoga helps in weight management, a brief discussion on weight management is imperative. A program aimed at achieving and/or maintaining a particular body weight is known as a weight management program. In general, this can be divided into two categories, weight gain and weight loss program.

Body Composition

The human body is composed of bones, lean muscle, fat, organs and water along with other parts such as skin, hair etc. Through a weight management program we aim to alter the body weight by altering either the lean muscle mass or the fat mass in the body. As is apparent the other constituent elements are not tampered with within the context of a weight management program. There are many methods to determine the amounts or percentages of different constituent elements in the body. Traditionally skin–fold measurements using calipers have been used for determining fat percentage. However, this method is slightly inaccurate and also does not provide a complete picture. Over the years numerous technologies have come into the forefront, which provide accurate and complete results in a matter of a few seconds. The commonly used ones include Ultrasound and Bio–electric Impedance Analysis.

Weight Loss versus weight gain

When the goal is to lose weight, the aim is to cut down on the fat mass. Fat is present in the body under the skin, also known as sub-cutaneous fat; and also around the organs predominantly in the abdominal region, this is known as visceral fat. When we lose fat, we lose it from all over the body and not from one targeted specific area. This is so because fat is an energy substrate that is used for metabolic purposes equal proportion from all areas of the body. The goal is to ensure that to meet the energy requirements of the body, whether it is for activities of daily life or for exercise, the energy is provided by burning the fat that is stored in the body. The goal is thus to lose weight by losing fat while maintaining or increasing lean muscle tissue.

When the goal is weight gain, the aim is to increase the lean muscle mass in the body and to cut down on the fat percentage. Gaining muscle mass is done through anabolic processes o growth processes. Lean muscle is gained through a combination of right exercise specifically resistance training along with the right kind of diet, which provides the body with the necessary fuel to grow. Contrary to weight loss, lean muscle tissue can be gained in specific areas of the body. By working out or exercising the muscles of the lower body, lean muscle tissue will be added to the muscle groups of the legs such as quadriceps, hamstrings and calves. By working out on the muscles of the upper body, lean muscle tissue will be added to the chest, shoulders, biceps, triceps and forearms. Within each of these muscle groups there are individual muscles that can be worked out by performing a whole variety of exercises. Except when a person is severely underweight with little fat in the body, generally fat is limited to a certain percentage. In a normal healthy male fat percentage should be around 10 – 15% while that in women it should be around 20 -25%. This is so because even fat has many important functions in the body such as thermo regulation, cushioning and protection of organs, and as an efficient energy store.

Healthy Weight Management

Healthy weight management is a multifaceted concept that is done in a gradual manner. The four pillars of wellness are physical exercise, diet & nutrition, rest & mental relaxation and attitude. Weight loss done in a way that ignores any particular aspect of wellness will invariably lead to sub-optimal results. For example, a weight management program that concentrates only on diet will help the individual to lose weight; but the weight loss thus achieved will include loss of lean muscle tissue as well which is undesirable.

Secondly, the rate at which weight loss or gain happens is also very important. In an effort to lose weight fast individuals get carried away at times and lose weight too fast. This is also not desired since the different systems of the body such as cardiovascular system, hormonal system etc. are used to functioning in a particular manner for the specific body type. Sudden changes are not well adapted by these systems as a result of which there are chances that some complications may arise. A good benchmark is loss or gain of 1 to 2 pounds of body weight per week. This gives time to the body to make necessary adjustments. Weight management done in this particular manner is considered healthy.

Yoga through different *asanas* that resemble body weighted exercises provides resistance training to different muscle groups. By performing particular *asanas* that target specific muscle groups we can increase the lean muscle tissue mass for muscles of that group. In such a way yoga can help in healthy weight gain that is through an increase in lean mass. In the following section though, the problem of weight loss has been catered to since the positive psychological effects that yoga has is applicable to weight gain programs in almost exactly the same way.

Benefits of yoga in relation to weight loss

One of the most widely accepted benefits of yoga is that it helps in healthy weight management. Not only does it work on the physical aspects of weight loss but also helps in tuning the mental faculties in a positive manner such that weight loss is facilitated. Since yoga promotes healthy weight loss, it is sustainable unlike unhealthy methods such as crash dieting.

Weight loss – background

A person can be overweight due to numerous reasons such as physiological, psychological, social and cultural factors. Whereas, certain lifestyle patterns are easier to alter leading to weight loss, there are other physiological parameters such as hormonal issues and psychological parameters such as emotional issues like depression and anxiety disorders; these may pose significantly greater problems in achieving weight loss. These emotional complications lead to people having literally no control over their dietary habits, emotional eating may follow which leads to weight gain. Even those who go on strict dietary regimens like crash diets are prone to gaining the lost weight back again. Even if they see results for a while, it is highly probable that they lose focus at some time and the binge eating that follows causes them to gain back all the lost weight. Obesity can be chronic in which a person keeps gaining weight steadily and continuously; it can also be fluctuating in nature, wherein a person gains and looses weight in a fluctuating manner.

How Yoga works

As seen above, there are many reasons for a person gaining weight. Yoga is extremely efficient in weight loss since it provides a multi–faceted approach; it does not work on the symptoms alone, but targets the root cause or core of the problem. It takes into account physical, emotional and mental components in dealing with the problem. Losing weight through yoga involves improving cardiovascular endurance, detoxification, increasing the metabolic rate, improving focus and awareness of goals and attaining appropriate hormonal balance. Practice of certain forms of yoga which are extremely fast paced and vigorous in nature resembles a cardiovascular endurance workout. There is hardly any gap between two *asanas* or postures, as a result of which the heart rate increases and is maintained at these high levels during the entire session. In such a manner, forms of yoga such as *Power yoga* and *Bikram yoga* are more efficient in comparison to forms such as *Iyengar yoga*. Practice of *kriyas* such as *surya namaskar* and *kapal bhati* done at a fast pace provide a decent cardiovascular workout.

Through different *asanas* specific training of different parts of the body can be performed. It is believed that flexion of the trunk brings about a certain amount of calmness while extension of the trunk leads to boosting of energy in the body. Practice of *pranayama* leads to a reduction in anxiety, helps in detoxifying the body and also increases metabolism. It also helps in an increased capacity of the body to transport essential nutrients and oxygen to different parts of the body where they can be utilized effectively. Yoga also effects the secretion of hormones from the thyroid and pituitary glands, which brings about a balance in the hormonal system and consequently positively affects the metabolic rate. *Pranayama* and meditation provide a calming influence over the mind. There is an increase in awareness of the present and this helps in improving focus. In such a way yoga helps in increasing adherence to the weight loss program. It also enforces the link between mind & body. One becomes more aware of the present, of what is being eaten and when the body feels full. This understanding is important in creating an environment where healthy eating is promoted and is sustainable. It is not based on the fabric of denial, which is bound to fail either today or tomorrow.

Weight loss is a complex problem and therefore the solution cannot be one–dimensional. Just working on calorie intake or burning calories through intense long duration workouts will not provide a sustainable solution. Yoga on the contrary works in a holistic manner. The attempt is towards creating a harmony between mind, body & soul. The entire exercise is looked at positively rather than as a punishment through which the body needs to be put for attaining weight loss. It is the entire process of the present that becomes enjoyable and this positivity ensures weight loss results.

Precautions to be considered while performing Yoga

Yoga is an extremely safe practice. However, risks present themselves specifically when without adequate knowledge people start performing complex *asanas*. The following precautions need to be taken before beginning the practice of Yoga:

1. It is recommended to consult a doctor or physician before starting any kind of yogic practice in case of severe conditions of osteoporosis, spine related problems, hypertension and also in case of pregnancy.

2. It is highly recommended that yoga be learnt under the supervision of a learned instructor. It may seem easy to follow books and online tutorials, but if improperly performed may be risky.

3. Understand your body and know the limits to which it can be

stretched. The body should not be pushed to an extent where chances of injury become high. For example there may be a slight discomfort such as a mild stretch that may be experienced while performing a particular *asana*; this is fine. However, there should be no pain whatsoever. In case this happens then it is highly recommended to stop immediately before an injury occurs.

4. It is important to go slow and at a steady pace that is comfortable for the body. In group classes there is a tendency to push beyond acceptable limits, so that synchronization with the group is maintained. It is recommended that yoga should be practiced at a pace where one is comfortable. Since it is not a race, there is no reason why more time cannot be devoted to learning a particular aspect that may perhaps be difficult to grasp.

Yoga is not a pill that will provide instant results. It is a way of life; a holistic practice that improves all aspects of life and creates harmony between the body, mind and soul.

Body goals diary

_____

_____

_____

_____

_____

_____

_____

_____

_____

_____

_____

_____

_____

Body goals diary

_____

_____

_____

_____

_____

_____

_____

_____

_____

_____

_____

_____

_____

_____

Body goals diary

_____

_____

_____

_____

_____

_____

_____

_____

_____

_____

_____

_____

_____

_____

Body goals diary

_____

_____

_____

_____

_____

_____

_____

_____

_____

_____

_____

_____

_____

Body goals diary

_____

_____

_____

_____

_____

_____

_____

_____

_____

_____

_____

_____

_____

Body goals diary

_____

_____

_____

_____

_____

_____

_____

_____

_____

_____

_____

_____

_____

Body goals diary

_____

_____

_____

_____

_____

_____

_____

_____

_____

_____

_____

_____

_____

Body goals diary

_____

_____

_____

_____

_____

_____

_____

_____

_____

_____

_____

_____

_____

Body goals diary

_____

_____

_____

_____

_____

_____

_____

_____

_____

_____

_____

_____

_____

_____

Body goals diary

_____

_____

_____

_____

_____

_____

_____

_____

_____

_____

_____

_____

_____

Body goals diary

_____

_____

_____

_____

_____

_____

_____

_____

_____

_____

_____

_____

_____

Body goals diary

_____

_____

_____

_____

_____

_____

_____

_____

_____

_____

_____

_____

_____

_____

Body goals diary

_____

_____

_____

_____

_____

_____

_____

_____

_____

_____

_____

_____

_____

_____

_____

Body goals diary

_____

_____

_____

_____

_____

_____

_____

_____

_____

_____

_____

_____

_____

Body goals diary

_____

_____

_____

_____

_____

_____

_____

_____

_____

_____

_____

_____

_____

_____

Body goals diary

_____

_____

_____

_____

_____

_____

_____

_____

_____

_____

_____

_____

Body goals diary

_____

_____

_____

_____

_____

_____

_____

_____

_____

_____

_____

_____

_____

Body goals diary

_____

_____

_____

_____

_____

_____

_____

_____

_____

_____

_____

_____

_____

Body goals diary

_____

_____

_____

_____

_____

_____

_____

_____

_____

_____

_____

_____

_____

Body goals diary

_____

_____

_____

_____

_____

_____

_____

_____

_____

_____

_____

_____

_____

About the author

C. T. Pam is not a physician, rather she is a regular person who has explored many avenues of eating healthy and finding a healthy lifestyle balance. After a car accident in 2010 left her unable to continue running, she found a work-life balance that has helped her maintain a healthy lifestyle. C. T. Pam has a B.A. in Political Science and Studio Art, an MBA with a entrepreneurship concentration and is currently pursuing a doctoral degree with a research focus in Entrepreneurship.

Book description

This book includes sound advice and facts regarding

- Introduction to weight management
- Choosing meal portions

While this book doesn't intend to tell the reader the best way to lead a healthy lifestyle, the author advises the reader to take away items that he or she can realistically achieve. You won't lose 50 pounds overnight, and you will have an opportunity to explore options that might benefit your physical, emotional and lifestyle needs. This book includes pages for the reader to record their goals and progress.

Volume 5 is an excerpt from Adopting a healthy lifestyle (1-884711-34-0)

Also available from Innovative Publishers

Introduction to the Paleo diet. (978-1884711466)

Introduction to the Paleo diet + 200 recipes (1884711820)

Love is... (978-1884711138)

Extreme Betrayal (978-1884711084)

Beware the Bumble Bee (978-1884711091)

Doing business with the U. S. government (978-1884711107)

Visit http://innovative-publishers.com for ordering information

Find us online @

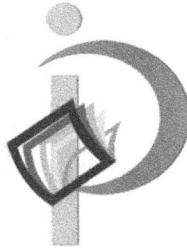

Innovative Publishers

InnovaPub

www.innovative-publishers.com

pub@innovative-publishers.com

http://innovativepublishers.blogspot.com/

http://www.facebook.com/InnovativePublishers

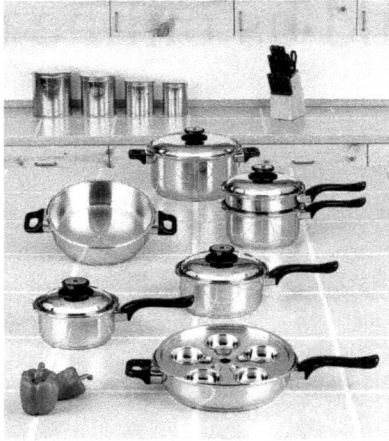

World's Finest™ 7-Ply Steam Control™ 17pc T304 Stainless Steel Cookware Set

Each piece is constructed of extra-heavy stainless steel and guaranteed to last a lifetime. Steam control valves make "waterless" cooking easy and the 7-ply construction spreads heat quickly and evenly, allowing one stack to cook. Cookware is also equipped with superbly styled phenolic handles resistant to heat, cold and detergents. Comes with a limited lifetime warranty. White box.

Suggested Retail Price : $2195.00

Item Number : GGKT17ULTRA

Set Contents

- 1.7Qt Covered Saucepan
- 2.5Qt Covered Saucepan
- 3.2Qt Covered Saucepan
- 7.5Qt Covered Roaster
- 11-3/8" Skillet, Double Boiler Unit With Capsule Bottom That You Can Also Use As An Extra 3Qt Saucepan
- 5 Egg Cups
- 5 Hole Utility Rack And High Dome Cover With Capsule Bottom So You Can Use As A Frypan
- Cover Fits Skillet Or Roaster

Features

- Extra-Heavy Stainless Steel Construction
- Heat-Resistant Phenolic Handles
- 7-Ply Construction

Limited Lifetime Warranty

» Estimated Case Weight : 36.55 Lbs.

Advertisement   64

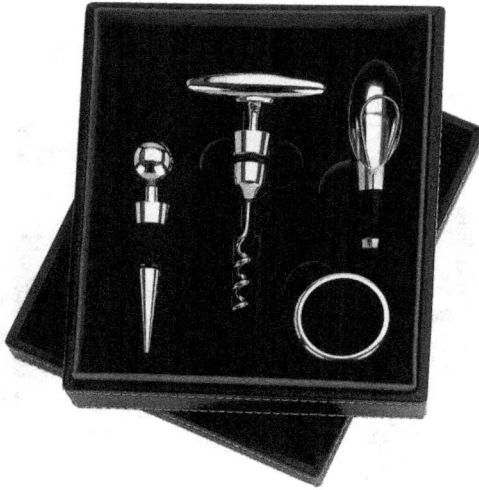

Wyndham House™ 4pc Wine Set in Storage Case

Wyndham House™ wine sets are a great compliment to any home bar, and are sure to add to the ease and elegance of wine presentations. Includes stainless steel wine spout, stainless steel wine ring, zinc alloy screw opener, and zinc alloy wine stopper. All enclosed in a 6-3/8" x 5-5/8" x 2-1/4" faux leather case.

Suggested Retail Price : $32.95

Next Ship Date : 01/05/2013

Item Number : GGKTWINE4

Features

- Stainless Steel Wine Spout
- Stainless Steel Wine Ring
- Zinc Alloy Screw Opener
- Zinc Alloy Wine Stopper
- 6-3/8" X 5-5/8" X 2-1/4" Faux Leather Case

Shipping Details

» Estimated Piece Weight : 1.10 Lbs.

 Advertisement

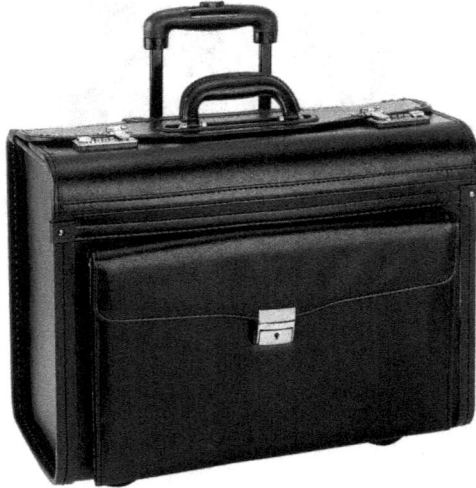

Embassy™ Sample/Pilot Case with Aluminum Trolley

Features PVC matte black exterior, rolling wheels, gunmetal combination locks, carrying handle, 2 exterior pockets, interior dividers, interior pockets, and pen holders. Measures 19" x 14" x 9".

Suggested Retail Price : $233.95

Number : BCPILOT3

Features

- Pvc Matte Black Exterior
- Rolling Wheels
- Gunmetal Combination Locks
- Carrying Handle
- 2 Exterior Side Pockets
- Interior Dividers & Pockets
- Pen Holders
- Measures 18" X 13" X 8"

Shipping Details

» Estimated Piece Weight : 8.70 Lbs.

To order products, go to the Innovative Publishers website and click Client specials. Clients receive up to 70% off the suggested retail price.

www.ingramcontent.com/pod-product-compliance
Lightning Source LLC
Chambersburg PA
CBHW050605280326
41933CB00011B/1995